FERTILITY DIET BIBLE FOR WOMEN OVER 30

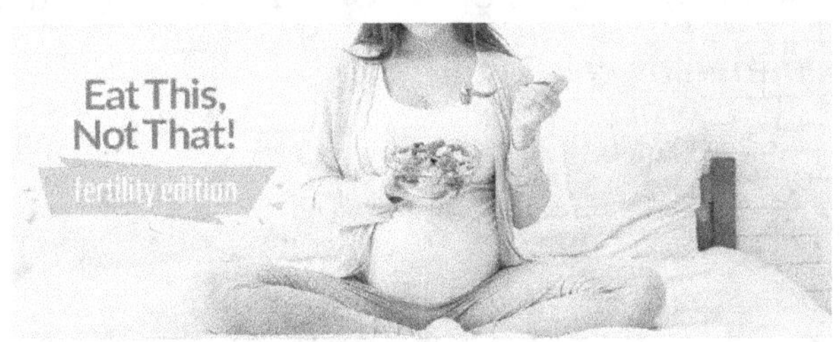

Fertility Diet Bible For Women, With Delicious Recipes, Tailored Meal Plan, And Effective Exercises To Boost Fertility.

Diana Courtney

Copyright © 2023 by Diana Courtney

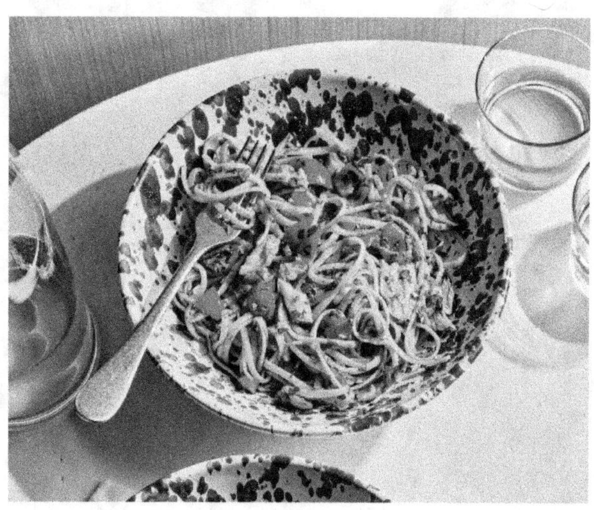

Table Of Content

INTRODUCTION

I am a dedicated nutritionist, intrigued by the rising concern of fertility in women especially those over 30 to 40 years of age. I made a passionate journey of research and experimentation, tirelessly studying different texts and herbal remedies. After months of dedication, I stumbled upon a recipe book in a colleagues library, filled with fertility-enhancing recipes and herbs. With excitement, I began combining traditional herbs and modern nutritional knowledge to create specialized meals to boost fertility and conception in women over 30.

With success in my discovery

I created this book to guide you through the journey to motherhood with delightful fertility recipes and herbs designed specifically for women over 30. Infused with essential nutrients and fertility-boosting ingredients to support your reproductive health and empower you to create a culinary path towards a joyful and healthy conception.

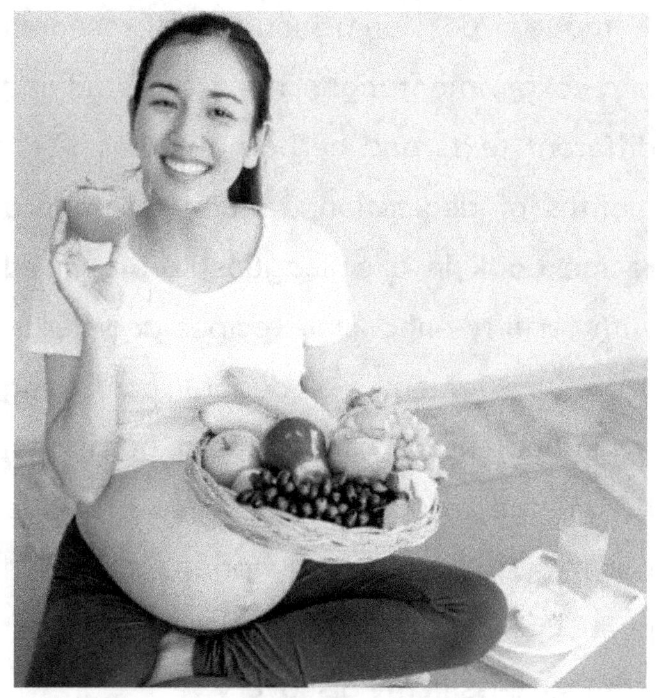

CHAPTER 1

Understanding Fertility and Aging

Fertility refers to the ability to conceive, and it gradually declines with age, especially for women. As women age, their ovarian reserve decreases, leading to reduced egg quantity and quality. This makes conception more challenging and increases the risk of infertility. Early awareness and timely consultation can aid in family planning.

The Impact of Age on Fertility:

Age has a significant impact on fertility in women. Fertility refers to a woman's ability to conceive and carry a pregnancy to term successfully. Here's how age affects fertility:

Peak Fertility in Early Adulthood: Women are most fertile in their early adulthood, typically in their 20s and early 30s. During this time, they have a higher number of healthy and viable eggs, and the chances of conception are at their highest.

Decline in Fertility after 30: As women age, their fertility gradually declines. After the age of 30 this decline becomes pronounced. The quality and quantity of a woman's eggs diminish, leading to reduced chances of conception. This decline accelerates as a woman approaches her mid-30s.

Increased Risk of Pregnancy Complications: As women get older, they face a higher risk of pregnancy complications, such as gestational diabetes, preeclampsia, and chromosomal abnormalities in the fetus (e.g., Down syndrome). In addition, the risk of miscarriage increases with age.

Decline in Ovarian Reserve: Ovarian reserve refers to the number of eggs a woman has left in her ovaries. The ovarian reserves decrease as the woman ages. This not only affects the chances of conception but also makes it challenging for older women to respond to fertility treatments like in vitro fertilization (IVF).

Menopause: Menopause is the stage when a woman's menstrual cycles stop, indicating the end of her reproductive years. The occurrence of Menopause is usually in the late 40s or early 50s. As women approach menopause, their fertility declines sharply until they can no longer conceive naturally.

Assisted Reproductive Technologies (ART): While age-related fertility decline cannot be entirely overcome, assisted reproductive technologies like IVF can help some older women conceive. However, success rates for ART also decline with age.

Optimizing Fertility Through Nutrition:

Optimizing fertility through nutrition is an essential aspect for women over 30 who are planning to conceive. Here are guidelines to consider:

Balanced Diet: Ensure you have a well-balanced diet that includes a variety of whole foods, such as fruits, vegetables, whole grains, lean proteins, and healthy fats. This helps provide essential nutrients necessary for reproductive health.

Folate and Folic Acid: Adequate folate intake is crucial during the preconception period and early pregnancy. It ensures birth defects in the baby's spinal cord and brain are prevented. Foods rich in folate include leafy greens, lentils, beans, fortified cereals, and avocados.

Iron: Iron is essential for red blood cell production and can prevent anemia, which may affect fertility. Good sources of iron include lean red meat, poultry, fish, beans, lentils, spinach, and fortified cereals.

Omega-3 Fatty Acids: Omega-3s play a role in hormone production and help regulate the menstrual cycle. They can be found in fatty fish (like salmon and sardines), chia seeds, flaxseeds, and walnuts.

Calcium and Vitamin D: These nutrients are important for bone health and may play a role in fertility. Dairy products, fortified plant-based milk, and sunlight exposure (for vitamin D) can help meet these needs.

Avoid Trans Fats: Trans fats are unhealthy fats found in processed and fried foods. They may increase the risk of ovulatory infertility. I would rather advice you pick healthy fats like olive oil, avocado oil, and nuts.

Limit Caffeine and Alcohol: High caffeine and alcohol intake may adversely affect fertility. Consider reducing their consumption while trying to conceive.

Stay Hydrated: Drink plenty of water to stay hydrated, as it can support overall health and fertility.

Maintain a Healthy Weight: Being either underweight or overweight can impact fertility. Strive to maintain a healthy weight through proper nutrition and regular physical activity.

Consider Supplementation: It can be challenging to get all the necessary nutrients from diet alone. Consult with a healthcare professional to assess if you need any additional supplements like prenatal vitamins.

Manage Stress: Chronic stress can affect hormone levels and ovulation. Engage in stress-reducing activities like yoga, meditation, or hobbies you enjoy.

Regular Exercise: Moderate and consistent physical activity can improve overall health and fertility. Avoid excessive or intense exercise that might disrupt menstrual cycles.

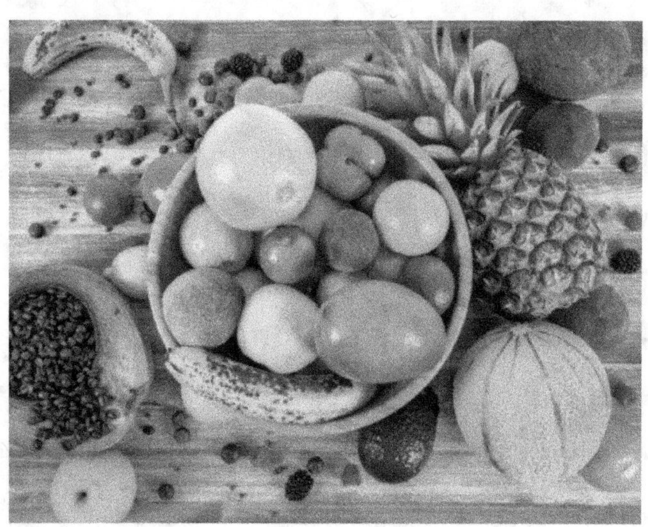

CHAPTER 2:

Building A Fertility-Friendly Diet

Building a fertility-friendly diet for women over 30 involves focusing on nutrients that support reproductive health and overall well-being. As women age, their fertility may decline, so it becomes essential to pay attention to the foods they consume. Here are some dietary guidelines to consider:

Key Nutrients for Fertility:

Maintaining proper nutrition is crucial for overall health and fertility, especially for women over 30 who may face age-related challenges when trying to conceive. While individual needs may vary, here are some key nutrients that play important roles in supporting fertility:

Folic Acid (Folate): Folic acid is essential for preventing neural tube defects in the developing fetus. It is recommended that women of childbearing age, including those over 30, consume 400 to 800 micrograms of folic acid daily.

Iron: Iron is important for healthy blood production and circulation, which is vital during pregnancy. Women over 30 should ensure they get enough iron in their diet or through supplements if recommended by a healthcare provider.

Omega-3 Fatty Acids: Omega-3s, especially DHA (docosahexaenoic acid), are important for brain development in babies and may also support fertility by promoting healthy hormone levels and reducing inflammation.

Calcium and Vitamin D: Calcium is essential for bone health and nerve function, while vitamin D helps with calcium absorption. Adequate levels of these nutrients are important for both the mother and the baby during pregnancy.

Zinc: Zinc is involved in various reproductive processes and may have a positive impact on egg quality and implantation.

Vitamin C and Vitamin E: These antioxidants can help protect eggs from oxidative stress and may improve overall reproductive health.

B Vitamins: B vitamins play various roles in the body, including supporting energy metabolism and reducing the risk of birth defects.

Coenzyme Q10 (CoQ10): Some research suggests that CoQ10 may improve egg quality and support fertility in women over 30.

Selenium: Selenium is an antioxidant that may play a role in protecting eggs and supporting overall fertility.

Magnesium: Magnesium is involved in numerous biochemical reactions in the body and may support reproductive health.

Foods to Include and Avoid:

When it comes to fertility, a balanced and nutritious diet can play a crucial role, especially for women over 30 who may face certain age-related fertility challenges. While no specific diet can guarantee pregnancy, incorporating certain foods and avoiding others can support overall reproductive health. Here are some dietary recommendations for women over 30 who are trying to conceive:

Foods to Include:

Fruits and Vegetables: Include a variety of colorful fruits and vegetables as they provide essential vitamins, minerals, and antioxidants that support reproductive health.

Whole Grains: Opt for whole grains like brown rice, quinoa, oats, and whole wheat, which are rich in fiber and nutrients, aiding hormonal balance.

Healthy Fats intake: avocados, nuts, seeds, and olive oil all these are sources of healthy fats. These fats are essential for hormone production and overall reproductive health.

Lean Proteins: Choose lean sources of protein like fish, poultry, beans, lentils, and tofu, which provide amino acids necessary for hormone regulation.

Dairy or Alternatives: Incorporate dairy products or fortified plant-based alternatives like almond milk, soy milk, or coconut milk to ensure an adequate intake of calcium and vitamin D.

Omega-3 Fatty Acids: Include fatty fish (salmon, mackerel, sardines) or flaxseeds and chia seeds, which are rich in omega-3 fatty acids that support reproductive function.

Iron-Rich Foods: Include iron-rich foods like spinach, lentils, beans, and lean red meat to support healthy blood levels and prevent anemia.

Folate-Rich Foods: Consume foods rich in folate, such as leafy greens, citrus fruits, beans, and fortified cereals. Folate is essential for fetal development.

Foods to Avoid or Limit:

Caffeine: Limit caffeine intake as high amounts may be associated with reduced fertility. Stick to moderate amounts of coffee, tea, or opt for decaffeinated versions.

Alcohol: It is advisable to limit alcohol consumption, as excessive alcohol intake can affect fertility and pregnancy.

Trans Fats: Avoid foods high in trans fats, such as processed and fried foods, as they may contribute to inflammation and hormonal imbalances.

High-Mercury Fish: Limit the consumption of high-mercury fish like swordfish, king mackerel, and tilefish, as mercury can negatively impact fertility and fetal development.

Added Sugars and Processed Foods: Reduce the intake of added sugars and heavily processed foods, as they may lead to weight gain and disrupt hormonal balance.

Soy Products: While moderate amounts of soy products are generally safe, it's best to limit highly processed soy foods as they contain compounds that may interfere with hormones.

Excessive Dieting: Avoid extreme or restrictive diets, as they can disrupt menstrual cycles and reduce fertility.

CHAPTER 3:

Breakfast Recipes:

Here are some nutrient-rich breakfast ideas that could potentially support women's health and fertility:

RECIPE 1: Berry and Yogurt Parfait:

Ingredients:

Greek yogurt,

mixed berries (blueberries, strawberries, raspberries),

honey,

granola.

Preparation: Layer yogurt, berries, and granola in a glass, drizzle honey on top.

Fertility Benefits: Rich in antioxidants, vitamins, and probiotics.

RECIPE 2: Chia Seed Pudding:

Ingredients:

Chia seeds,

almond milk,

honey,

fresh fruits (e.g., mango, kiwi).

Preparation: Mix chia seeds with almond milk and honey, refrigerate overnight, top with fresh fruits.

Fertility Benefits: Chia seeds are a good source of omega-3 fatty acids and fiber.

RECIPE 3: Spinach and Mushroom Omelette:

Ingredients:

Eggs,

spinach,

mushrooms,

onions,

olive oil,

salt,

pepper.

Preparation: Whisk eggs, sauté vegetables in olive oil, add eggs, cook until set.

Fertility Benefits: Rich in folate, iron, and vitamin D.

RECIPE 4: Whole Grain Banana Pancakes:

Ingredients:

Whole grain flour,

mashed bananas,

eggs,

milk,

baking powder.

Preparation: Mix ingredients, cook pancakes on a griddle.

Fertility Benefits: Whole grains offer complex carbs and bananas provide vitamins and minerals.

RECIPE 5: Avocado Toast:

Ingredients:

Whole grain bread,

avocado,

cherry tomatoes,

lemon juice,

salt,

pepper.

Preparation: Mash avocado, spread on toast, top with sliced tomatoes, lemon juice, salt, and pepper.

Fertility Benefits: Avocado is a good source of healthy fats and folate.

RECIPE 6: Salmon and Avocado Sandwich:

Ingredients:

Whole grain bread,

canned salmon,

avocado,

spinach,

lemon juice.

Preparation: Assemble ingredients into a sandwich.

Fertility Benefits: Salmon is rich in omega-3 fatty acids and protein.

RECIPE 7: Mango and Coconut Smoothie:

Ingredients:

Fresh mango,

coconut milk,

Greek yogurt,

honey.

Preparation: Blend ingredients until smooth.

Fertility Benefits: Mango is rich in vitamins A and C, and coconut milk provides healthy fats.

RECIPE 8: Quinoa Breakfast Bowl:

Ingredients:

Cooked quinoa,

mixed berries,

nuts (e.g., almonds, walnuts),

honey.

Preparation: Mix quinoa, berries, and nuts in a bowl, drizzle honey on top.

Fertility Benefits: Quinoa is a good source of protein and essential nutrients.

RECIPE 9: Blueberry Almond Overnight Oats:

Ingredients:

Rolled oats,

almond milk,

blueberries,

almond slices,

honey.

Preparation: Mix oats, almond milk, and blueberries, refrigerate overnight, top with almond slices and honey.

Fertility Benefits: Blueberries provide antioxidants and almonds offer healthy fats.

RECIPE 10: Pumpkin Seed Granola:

Ingredients:

Rolled oats,

pumpkin seeds,

honey,

coconut oil,

dried cranberries.

Preparation: Mix oats, pumpkin seeds, honey, and melted coconut oil, bake until golden, add dried cranberries.

Fertility Benefits: Pumpkin seeds are rich in zinc and iron.

RECIPE 11: Egg and Vegetable Breakfast Burrito:

Ingredients:

Whole wheat tortilla,

eggs,

bell peppers,

onions,

black beans,

salsa.

Preparation: Scramble eggs, sauté vegetables, assemble into a burrito with black beans and salsa.

Fertility Benefits: Black beans offer folate and fiber.

RECIPE 12: Pomegranate and Walnut Yogurt Bowl:

Ingredients:

Greek yogurt,

pomegranate seeds,

walnuts,

honey.

Preparation: Mix ingredients in a bowl.

Fertility Benefits: Pomegranate seeds are rich in antioxidants, and walnuts provide omega-3 fatty acids.

RECIPE 13: Sesame and Flaxseed Smoothie:

Ingredients:

Almond milk,

banana,

sesame seeds,

flaxseeds,

honey.

Preparation: Blend ingredients until smooth.

Fertility Benefits: Flaxseeds are a good source of omega-3 fatty acids and fiber.

RECIPE 14: Greek Frittata:

Ingredients:

Eggs,

spinach, feta cheese,

cherry tomatoes,

olive oil,

salt, and pepper.

Preparation: Whisk eggs, mix with spinach, feta, and tomatoes, bake until set.

Fertility Benefits: Spinach and tomatoes provide vitamins and antioxidants.

RECIPE 15: Ricotta and Berry Stuffed Crepes:

Ingredients:

Crepes (store-bought or homemade), ricotta cheese,

mixed berries,

honey.

Preparation: Spread ricotta and berries on crepes, drizzle honey, roll them up.

Fertility Benefits: Ricotta cheese offers protein and calcium.

RECIPE 16: Almond Butter and Banana Toast:

Ingredients:

Whole grain bread,

almond butter,

sliced bananas,

honey.

Preparation: Spread almond butter on toast, top with banana slices and honey.

Fertility Benefits: Almond butter provides healthy fats and bananas offer vitamins.

RECIPE 17: Asparagus and Tomato Frittata:

Ingredients:

Eggs,

asparagus,

cherry tomatoes,

onion,

olive oil,

salt, and pepper.

Preparation: Whisk eggs, sauté vegetables in olive oil, add eggs, cook until set.

Fertility Benefits: Asparagus is rich in folate and vitamin K.

RECIPE 18: Coconut and Almond Chia Pudding:

Ingredients:

Chia seeds,

coconut milk,

almond extract,

shredded coconut,

slivered almonds.

Preparation: Mix chia seeds, coconut milk, and almond extract, refrigerate overnight, top with shredded coconut and slivered almonds.

Fertility Benefits: Coconut milk and almonds offer healthy fats.

RECIPE 19: Green Smoothie Bowl:

Ingredients:

Spinach,

kale,

banana,

pineapple,

coconut water,

chia seeds.

Preparation: Blend ingredients until smooth, pour into a bowl, top with chia seeds.

Fertility Benefits: Leafy greens provide folate and other essential nutrients.

RECIPE 20: Sweet Potato Hash:

Ingredients:

Sweet potatoes,

bell peppers,

onions,

olive oil,

paprika,

salt, and pepper.

Preparation: Dice and sauté sweet potatoes, bell peppers, and onions in olive oil, season with paprika, salt, and pepper.

Fertility Benefits: Sweet potatoes are rich in beta-carotene and vitamin C.

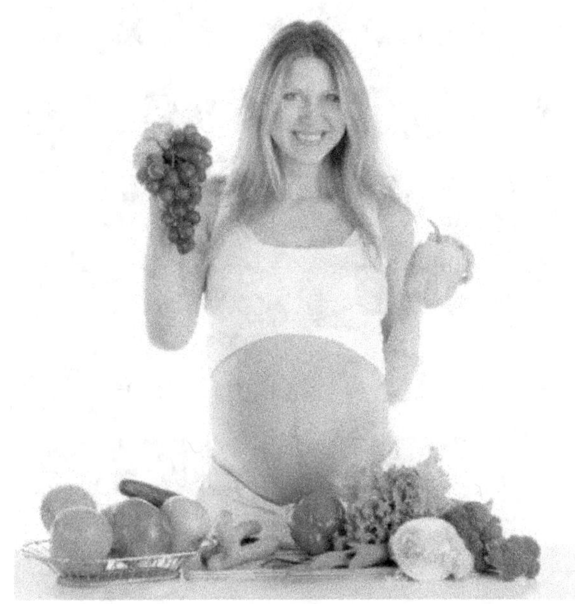

Best foods to boost fertility in females

Asparagus	Leafy greens
Seaweed	Fenugreek
Maca root	Sweet potatoes
Carrots	Cooked tomatoes
Broccoli	Beans and lentils
Garlic	Cinnamon
Extra virgin olive oil	Carbohydrates
Quinoa	Avocados
Bananas	Beets
Berries	Figs
Pomegranate	Citrus fruits

CHAPTER 4:

Lunch Recipes:

lunch recipes with ingredients, preparation instructions, and potential fertility benefits for women over 30:

RECIPE 1: Grilled Salmon Salad:

Ingredients:

Fresh salmon filet

Mixed greens (spinach, kale, arugula)

Cherry tomatoes

Avocado

Lemon juice

Olive oil

Salt and pepper

Preparation: Grill the salmon and toss it with mixed greens, cherry tomatoes, and sliced avocado. Dress the salad with lemon juice, olive oil, salt, and pepper.

Fertility Benefits: Salmon is rich in omega-3 fatty acids, which are essential for hormone production and reproductive health.

RECIPE 2: Quinoa and Vegetable Stir-fry:

Ingredients:

Quinoa

Broccoli

Bell peppers

Carrots

Snap peas

Garlic

Ginger

Soy sauce

Preparation: Cook quinoa according to package instructions. Stir-fry chopped vegetables with garlic and ginger in a bit of olive oil. Add cooked quinoa and soy sauce.

Fertility Benefits: Quinoa provides complex carbohydrates, while vegetables offer essential vitamins and minerals for overall health and fertility.

RECIPE 3: Chickpea and Spinach Curry:

Ingredients:

Chickpeas

Fresh spinach

Tomatoes

Onion

Garlic

Ginger

Coconut milk

Curry spices (turmeric, cumin, coriander)

Preparation: Sauté onion, garlic, and ginger. Add chopped tomatoes and simmer until soft. Stir in chickpeas, spinach, coconut milk, and curry spices. Cook until heated through.

Fertility Benefits: Chickpeas are a good source of plant-based protein and fiber, while spinach is rich in iron and other nutrients beneficial for fertility.

RECIPE 4: Lentil and Sweet Potato Soup:

Ingredients:

Red lentils

Sweet potatoes

Celery

Carrots

Vegetable broth

Turmeric

Cumin

Paprika

Preparation: Boil lentils and diced sweet potatoes in vegetable broth. Sauté celery and carrots, then add to the pot. Season with turmeric, cumin, and paprika.

Fertility Benefits: Lentils are rich in folate, a crucial nutrient for women trying to conceive. Sweet potatoes contain beta-carotene, which may improve fertility.

RECIPE 5: Whole Grain Pasta with Pesto:

Ingredients:

Whole grain pasta

Fresh basil

Pine nuts

Garlic

Parmesan cheese

Olive oil

Salt and pepper

Preparation: Cook whole grain pasta until al dente. Blend basil, pine nuts, garlic, parmesan cheese, and olive oil to make the pesto. Toss with pasta.

Fertility Benefits: Whole grain pasta offers complex carbs, and basil contains anti-inflammatory properties, which may support reproductive health.

RECIPE 6: Greek Quinoa Salad:

Ingredients:

Cooked quinoa

Cucumber

Cherry tomatoes

Red onion

Kalamata olives

Feta cheese

Lemon juice

Olive oil

Oregano

Preparation: Combine quinoa, diced cucumber, halved cherry tomatoes, sliced red onion, olives, and crumbled feta cheese. Dress with lemon juice, olive oil, and oregano.

Fertility Benefits: Quinoa provides essential nutrients, and the salad is rich in antioxidants and healthy fats from olives and olive oil.

RECIPE 7: Turkey and Vegetable Wrap:

Ingredients:

Whole grain tortilla wrap

Turkey slices

Avocado

Baby spinach

Shredded carrots

Hummus

Preparation: Spread hummus on the tortilla wrap. Layer turkey slices, avocado, baby spinach, and shredded carrots. Roll up and enjoy.

Fertility Benefits: Whole grain tortillas offer complex carbs, while avocado provides healthy fats and folate, which is important for fertility.

RECIPE 8: Spinach and Mushroom Omelette:

Ingredients:

Eggs

Fresh spinach

Mushrooms

Onion

Olive oil

Salt and pepper

Preparation: Sauté sliced mushrooms and diced onion in olive oil. Beat eggs and pour them into the pan. Add fresh spinach. Cook until the eggs are set.

Fertility Benefits: Eggs are a good source of protein and essential nutrients like choline, which is important for fertility and fetal development.

RECIPE 9: Black Bean and Quinoa Burrito Bowl:

Ingredients:

Cooked quinoa

Black beans

Bell peppers

Corn kernels

Avocado

Salsa

Lime juice

Cilantro

Preparation: Combine quinoa, black beans, diced bell peppers, and corn kernels. Top with sliced avocado, salsa, lime juice, and chopped cilantro.

Fertility Benefits: Black beans provide protein and fiber, while quinoa offers essential nutrients for overall health and fertility.

RECIPE 10: Tofu and Broccoli Stir-fry:

Ingredients:

Firm tofu

Broccoli florets

Red bell pepper

Zucchini

Soy sauce

Sesame oil

Ginger

Preparation: Cube tofu and stir-fry with broccoli, red bell pepper, and zucchini. Season with soy sauce, sesame oil, and grated ginger.

Fertility Benefits: Tofu is a good source of plant-based protein, and the vegetables offer vitamins and minerals that promote reproductive health.

RECIPE 11: Mediterranean Chickpea Salad: Ingredients:

Chickpeas

Cucumber

Cherry tomatoes

Red onion

Kalamata olives

Feta cheese

Fresh parsley

Lemon juice

Olive oil

Preparation: Combine chickpeas, diced cucumber, halved cherry tomatoes, sliced red onion, olives, and crumbled feta cheese. Dress with lemon juice and olive oil. Garnish with fresh parsley.

Fertility Benefits: This salad is rich in plant-based protein, antioxidants, and healthy fats, supporting overall health and fertility.

RECIPE 12: Cauliflower Fried Rice:
Ingredients:

Cauliflower rice (grated cauliflower)

Eggs

Peas

Carrots

Scallions

Garlic

Soy sauce

Preparation: Stir-fry grated cauliflower with peas, diced carrots, chopped scallions, and minced garlic. Push the veggies to the side and scramble eggs in the pan. Mix everything together and add soy sauce.

Fertility Benefits: Cauliflower is low in carbs and provides essential nutrients, while the veggies offer vitamins and minerals that support fertility.

RECIPE 13: Baked Sweet Potato with Black Bean Chili:

Ingredients:

Sweet potatoes

Black beans

Diced tomatoes

Onion

Garlic

Chili powder

Cumin

Paprika

Preparation: Bake sweet potatoes until tender. Sauté onion and garlic. Add black beans, diced tomatoes, and spices. Simmer until the chili thickens. Serve over the baked sweet potatoes.

Fertility Benefits: Sweet potatoes provide nutrients like beta-carotene, while black beans offer protein and fiber for fertility support.

RECIPE 14: Avocado and Shrimp Salad:

Ingredients:

Avocado

Cooked shrimp

Mixed greens

Cherry tomatoes

Red onion

Lemon juice

Olive oil

Preparation: Slice avocado and toss it with cooked shrimp, mixed greens, halved cherry tomatoes, and thinly sliced red onion. Dress with lemon juice and olive oil.

Fertility Benefits: Shrimp is a good source of lean protein, and avocado offers healthy fats and folate, which is essential for fertility.

RECIPE 15: Stuffed Bell Peppers with Quinoa and Beans:

Ingredients:

Bell peppers

Cooked quinoa

Black beans

Corn kernels

Salsa

Shredded cheese

Preparation: Cut the tops off bell peppers and remove the seeds. Mix cooked quinoa, black beans, corn kernels, and salsa. Stuff the peppers with the mixture and top with shredded cheese. Bake until the peppers are tender.

Fertility Benefits: Bell peppers provide vitamin C, while quinoa and black beans offer essential nutrients for reproductive health.

RECIPE 16: Mediterranean Tuna Salad:

Ingredients:

Canned tuna (in water)

Cucumber

Cherry tomatoes

Red onion

Kalamata olives

Feta cheese

Fresh dill

Lemon juice

Olive oil

Preparation: Drain canned tuna and mix with diced cucumber, halved cherry tomatoes, sliced red onion, olives, crumbled feta cheese, and chopped dill. Dress with lemon juice and olive oil.

Fertility Benefits: Tuna offers protein and omega-3 fatty acids, while the salad provides antioxidants and healthy fats.

RECIPE 17: Mexican Quinoa Stuffed Peppers:

Ingredients:

Bell peppers

Cooked quinoa

Cooked black beans

Corn kernels

Diced tomatoes

Taco seasoning

Shredded cheese

Preparation: Cut the tops off bell peppers and remove the seeds. Mix cooked quinoa, black beans, corn kernels, diced tomatoes, and taco seasoning. Stuff the peppers with the mixture and top with shredded cheese. Bake until the peppers are tender.

Fertility Benefits: This recipe combines protein-rich quinoa and black beans with essential nutrients from the vegetables.

RECIPE 18: Eggplant and Chickpea Curry:

Ingredients:

Eggplant

Chickpeas

Onion

Garlic

Ginger

Tomatoes

Coconut milk

Curry spices (turmeric, cumin, coriander)

Preparation: Sauté onion, garlic, and ginger. Add diced eggplant and chopped tomatoes. Stir in chickpeas and coconut milk. Season with curry spices and simmer until the eggplant is tender.

Fertility Benefits: Eggplant provides antioxidants, while chickpeas and coconut milk offer nutrients that support reproductive health.

RECIPE 19: Green Goddess Salad with Grilled Chicken:

Ingredients:

Grilled chicken breast

Mixed greens (spinach, kale, arugula)

Cucumber

Avocado

Green goddess dressing (made from fresh herbs, yogurt, and lemon)

Preparation: Grill chicken breast and slice it. Toss mixed greens with sliced cucumber and diced avocado. Drizzle green goddess dressing over the salad and top with grilled chicken.

Fertility Benefits: This salad is rich in leafy greens, avocado, and lean protein from the grilled chicken.

RECIPE 20: Tomato Basil Mozzarella Sandwich:

Ingredients:

Whole grain bread

Sliced fresh mozzarella cheese

Tomato slices

Fresh basil leaves

Balsamic glaze

Preparation: Layer mozzarella cheese, tomato slices, and fresh basil leaves between two slices of whole grain bread. Drizzle balsamic glaze on the filling and grill or press the sandwich until the cheese melts.

Fertility Benefits: Whole grain bread provides complex carbs, while the sandwich offers essential nutrients from the mozzarella, tomatoes, and basil.

All these recipes include ingredients with potential fertility benefits.

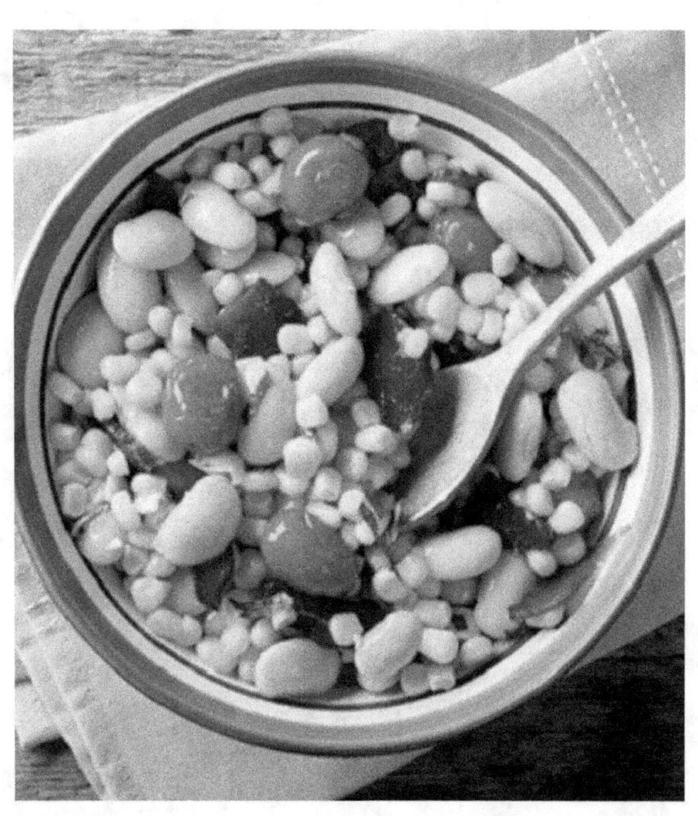

CHAPTER 5:

Dinner Recipes

These recipes focus on including ingredients that are generally considered beneficial for fertility

RECIPE 1: Grilled Salmon with Quinoa and Steamed Broccoli

Ingredients:

Salmon fillet

Quinoa

Broccoli

Preparation:

Grill the salmon fillet until cooked through.

Cook quinoa according to package instructions.

Steam the broccoli until tender. Serve together for a meal rich in omega-3 fatty acids, protein, and fiber, which can promote fertility and hormone balance.

RECIPE 2: Spinach and Mushroom Stuffed Chicken Breast

Ingredients:

Chicken breast

Spinach

Mushrooms

Olive oil

Preparation:

Preheat the oven to 375°F (190°C).

Sauté spinach and mushrooms in olive oil until wilted.

Cut a pocket into the chicken breast and stuff with the spinach and mushroom mixture.

Bake for 25-30 minutes until chicken is cooked through. This dish provides iron, folate, and other essential nutrients beneficial for fertility.

RECIPE 3: Lentil and Vegetable Stir-Fry

Ingredients:

Lentils

Assorted vegetables (carrots, bell peppers, zucchini, etc.)

Garlic

Soy sauce

Preparation:

Cook lentils according to package instructions.

Stir-fry chopped vegetables and garlic in a pan with soy sauce.

Mix in cooked lentils. Lentils are rich in folate and protein, while the veggies offer antioxidants and vitamins that support reproductive health.

RECIPE 4: Quinoa and Black Bean Salad

Ingredients:

Quinoa

Black beans

Red bell pepper

Cilantro

Lime juice

Preparation:

Cook quinoa according to package instructions.

Mix cooked quinoa with drained and rinsed black beans.

Add chopped red bell pepper, cilantro, and lime juice. This salad is loaded with plant-based protein, fiber, and folate, all of which are beneficial for fertility.

RECIPE 5: Beef and Sweet Potato Stir-Fry

Ingredients:

Lean beef strips

Sweet potatoes

Broccoli florets

Ginger

Soy sauce

Preparation:

Stir-fry beef in a pan until browned.

Add sliced sweet potatoes, broccoli, and ginger, and cook until tender.

Mix in soy sauce. Lean beef supplies iron and protein, while sweet potatoes offer vitamin A and fiber, supporting reproductive health.

RECIPE 6: Shrimp and Avocado Salad

Ingredients:

Shrimp

Avocado

Spinach

Cherry tomatoes

Balsamic vinaigrette dressing

Preparation:

Grill or cook the shrimp until pink and cooked through.

Assemble a salad with spinach, diced avocado, and cherry tomatoes.

Top with cooked shrimp and drizzle with balsamic vinaigrette. Shrimp is a good source of vitamin D, while avocados provide healthy fats and folate, all of which can enhance fertility.

RECIPE 7: Eggplant and Chickpea Curry

Ingredients:

Eggplant

Chickpeas

Coconut milk

Curry spices (turmeric, cumin, coriander)

Preparation:

Sauté eggplant in a pan until tender.

Add cooked chickpeas, coconut milk, and curry spices. Simmer until flavors meld. Eggplant supplies antioxidants, while chickpeas offer protein and fiber, making this curry fertility-friendly.

RECIPE 8: Baked Cod with Asparagus

Ingredients:

Cod fillets

Asparagus spears

Lemon

Olive oil

Preparation:

Preheat the oven to 400°F (200°C).

Place cod fillets and asparagus on a baking sheet.

Drizzle with olive oil and lemon juice.

Bake for 15-20 minutes or until fish is cooked. Cod is a good source of lean protein, and asparagus provides vitamins and antioxidants, supporting fertility.

RECIPE 9: Veggie and Tofu Stir-Fry

Ingredients:

Firm tofu

Assorted vegetables (broccoli, snow peas, carrots, etc.)

Ginger

Garlic

Soy sauce

Preparation:

Cut tofu into cubes and stir-fry in a pan until lightly browned.

Add chopped vegetables, ginger, and garlic, and stir-fry until tender-crisp.

Mix in soy sauce. Tofu offers plant-based protein, while the veggies provide vitamins and minerals crucial for fertility.

RECIPE 10: Baked Zucchini Boats with Ground Turkey

Ingredients:

Zucchini

Ground turkey

Onion

Tomato sauce

Preparation:

Preheat the oven to 375°F (190°C).

Cut zucchini in half lengthwise and scoop out the centers to create "boats."

Brown ground turkey with diced onions in a pan.

Stuff the zucchini boats with the turkey mixture and cover with tomato sauce.

Bake for 20-25 minutes until zucchini is tender. Ground turkey is a lean source of protein, and zucchini provides vitamins and antioxidants, making this dish fertility-friendly.

RECIPE 11: Pomegranate Glazed Chicken with Roasted Vegetables

Ingredients:

Chicken thighs

Pomegranate juice

Honey

Brussel sprouts

Carrots

Olive oil

Preparation:

Preheat the oven to 425°F (220°C).

In a saucepan, simmer pomegranate juice and honey until it thickens.

Brush the chicken thighs with the pomegranate glaze and roast in the oven.

Toss Brussel sprouts and carrots with olive oil, salt, and pepper, and roast until tender. Pomegranate juice is rich in antioxidants, and the roasted vegetables provide vitamins and fiber, supporting fertility.

RECIPE 12: Whole Wheat Pasta Primavera

Ingredients:

Whole wheat pasta

Broccoli

Bell peppers

Cherry tomatoes

Olive oil

Parmesan cheese

Preparation:

Cook whole wheat pasta according to package instructions.

Blanch broccoli florets, bell peppers, and halved cherry tomatoes in boiling water for a few minutes.

Toss the cooked pasta and vegetables with olive oil and top with grated Parmesan cheese. Whole wheat pasta offers complex carbohydrates and fiber, while the vegetables provide essential nutrients for fertility.

RECIPE 13: Stuffed Bell Peppers with Quinoa and Turkey

Ingredients:

Bell peppers

Ground turkey

Quinoa

Onion

Tomato sauce

Preparation:

Preheat the oven to 375°F (190°C).

Cut the tops off bell peppers and remove the seeds.

Sauté ground turkey and diced onions in a pan until cooked.

Cook quinoa according to package instructions.

Mix the cooked turkey and quinoa, stuff the bell peppers, and cover with tomato sauce.

Bake for 20-25 minutes until peppers are tender. Ground turkey supplies protein, while quinoa offers protein and fiber, making this a fertility-friendly dish.

RECIPE 14: Sardine and Tomato Stew

Ingredients:

Canned sardines

Tomatoes

Onion

Garlic

Red pepper flakes

Preparation:

Sauté diced onions and minced garlic in a pot until softened.

Add canned sardines and tomatoes to the pot, breaking the sardines into chunks.

Season with red pepper flakes and simmer for a few minutes until flavors meld. Sardines are an excellent source of omega-3 fatty acids and protein, promoting fertility and overall health.

RECIPE 15: Veggie Frittata

Ingredients:

Eggs

Spinach

Bell peppers

Onion

Feta cheese

Preparation:

Preheat the oven to 375°F (190°C).

Sauté chopped vegetables in a pan until tender.

In a bowl, whisk eggs and mix in the sautéed vegetables and crumbled feta cheese.

Pour the mixture into a greased baking dish and bake for 20-25 minutes until set.

Eggs supply high-quality protein, while spinach and bell peppers offer vitamins and minerals crucial for fertility.

RECIPE 16: Quinoa Stuffed Portobello Mushrooms

Ingredients:

Portobello mushrooms

Quinoa

Kale

Goat cheese

Preparation:

Preheat the oven to 375°F (190°C).

Cook quinoa according to package instructions.

Sauté chopped kale until wilted.

Mix cooked quinoa and kale together and stuff into the Portobello mushrooms.

Top with crumbled goat cheese.

Bake for 15-20 minutes until mushrooms are tender. This dish combines the fertility benefits of quinoa, kale, and goat cheese in a delicious way.

RECIPE 17: Baked Sweet Potatoes with Chickpea and Kale Salad

Ingredients:

Sweet potatoes

Chickpeas

Kale

Lemon juice

Tahini

Preparation:

Preheat the oven to 400°F (200°C).

Pierce sweet potatoes with a fork and bake until tender.

Mix drained and rinsed chickpeas with chopped kale, lemon juice, and tahini to make a salad. Serve the baked sweet potatoes topped with the chickpea and kale salad for a nutrient-packed meal.

RECIPE 18: Tofu and Vegetable Curry

Ingredients:

Firm tofu

Assorted vegetables (cauliflower, peas, carrots, etc.)

Coconut milk

Curry spices (turmeric, cumin, coriander)

Preparation:

Cut tofu into cubes and sauté in a pan until lightly browned.

Add chopped vegetables and sauté until tender-crisp.

Stir in coconut milk and curry spices, and simmer until flavors blend. This plant-based curry is rich in protein, vitamins, and antioxidants, supporting fertility.

RECIPE 19: Shrimp and Quinoa Bowl with Avocado Dressing

Ingredients:

Shrimp

Quinoa

Avocado

Lime juice

Greek yogurt

Cilantro

Preparation:

Grill or cook the shrimp until pink and cooked through.

Cook quinoa according to package instructions.

Blend avocado, lime juice, Greek yogurt, and cilantro to make a creamy dressing.

Assemble a bowl with cooked quinoa, shrimp, and drizzle with the avocado dressing. This bowl is loaded with protein, healthy fats, and fertility-enhancing nutrients.

RECIPE 20: Brown Rice and Vegetable Stir-Fry with Cashews

Ingredients:

Brown rice

Assorted vegetables (broccoli, carrots, bell peppers, etc.)

Cashews

Soy sauce

Preparation:

Cook brown rice according to package instructions.

Stir-fry chopped vegetables in a pan until tender-crisp.

Mix in cooked brown rice and cashews, and add soy sauce for seasoning. This stir-fry is rich in fiber, vitamins, and minerals, supporting fertility and overall health.

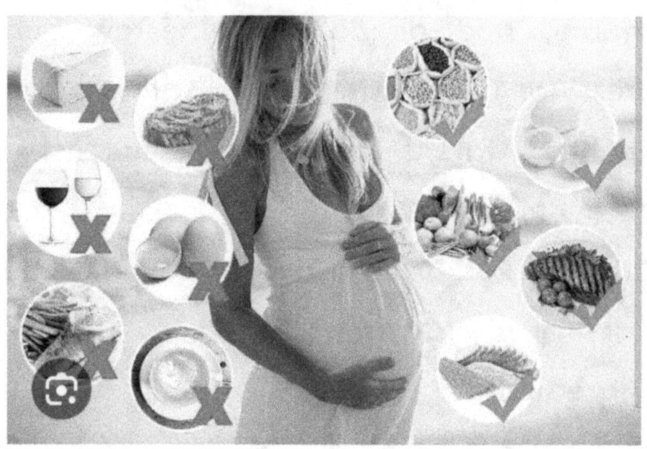

CHAPTER 6:

Snack Recipes:

These snacks can support reproductive health in women over 30.

RECIPE 1: Chia Seed Pudding:

Ingredients:

2 tbsp chia seeds

1 cup almond milk

1 teaspoon honey

Fresh berries (blueberries, strawberries, etc.)

Preparation: Mix chia seeds, almond milk, and honey. Refrigerate for at least 2 hours. Top with fresh berries rich in antioxidants.

Fertility Benefits: Chia seeds contain omega-3 fatty acids, fiber, and protein, which support hormone balance and reproductive health.

RECIPE 2: Avocado Toast:

Ingredients:

1 ripe avocado

Whole-grain bread

Lemon juice

Chili flakes (optional)

Preparation: Mash the avocado with lemon juice. Spread it on whole-grain toast and sprinkle chili flakes for added flavor.

Fertility Benefits: Avocados are a great source of healthy fats, folate, and vitamin E, which can support fertility.

RECIPE 3: Greek Yogurt Parfait:

Ingredients:

1 cup Greek yogurt

Mixed nuts and seeds (almonds, walnuts, pumpkin seeds)

Fresh fruits (kiwi, pomegranate seeds)

Preparation: Layer Greek yogurt, nuts, seeds, and fresh fruits in a glass to make a delicious parfait.

Fertility Benefits: Greek yogurt provides calcium, while nuts and seeds offer essential fatty acids and minerals beneficial for fertility.

RECIPE 4: Salmon Cucumber Bites:

Ingredients:

Smoked salmon slices

Cucumber slices

Dill sprigs

Cream cheese (optional)

Preparation: Top each cucumber slice with smoked salmon, a small dollop of cream cheese, and a dill sprig.

Fertility Benefits: Salmon is rich in omega-3 fatty acids and protein, which can promote reproductive health.

RECIPE 5: Berry Spinach Smoothie:

Ingredients:

1 cup spinach

1 cup mixed berries (strawberries, blueberries, raspberries)

1 banana

1 cup almond milk

1 tbsp flax seeds

Preparation: Blend all the ingredients until smooth.

Fertility Benefits: This smoothie packs a punch of antioxidants, vitamins, and minerals that support overall health and fertility.

RECIPE 6: Quinoa Salad:

Ingredients:

Cooked quinoa

Cherry tomatoes

Cucumber

Red bell pepper

Feta cheese

Olive oil and lemon dressing

Preparation: Mix all the ingredients with the dressing.

Fertility Benefits: Quinoa is a protein-rich grain, and the colorful veggies provide essential nutrients and antioxidants.

RECIPE 7: Hard-Boiled Eggs with Hummus:

Ingredients:

Hard-boiled eggs

Hummus

Carrot sticks

Preparation: Serve hard-boiled eggs with a side of hummus and carrot sticks.

Fertility Benefits: Eggs are a good source of protein and choline, while hummus provides healthy fats and fiber.

RECIPE 8: Sesame Edamame:

Ingredients:

Steamed edamame

Toasted sesame seeds

Sea salt

Preparation: Toss steamed edamame with sesame seeds and a pinch of sea salt.

Fertility Benefits: Edamame is a rich source of plant-based protein, fiber, and iron.

RECIPE 9: Fertility Trail Mix:

Ingredients:

Almonds

Cashews

Pumpkin seeds

Dried cherries

Dark chocolate chips

Preparation:

Mix all the ingredients to make your trail mix.

Fertility Benefits: Nuts and seeds offer a variety of nutrients like zinc, selenium, and vitamin E that support fertility.

RECIPE 10: Cottage Cheese with Pineapple:

Ingredients:

Low-fat cottage cheese

Fresh pineapple chunks

Preparation: Top cottage cheese with fresh pineapple chunks.

Fertility Benefits: Pineapple contains bromelain, an enzyme believed to have anti-inflammatory properties that may benefit fertility.

RECIPE 11: Stuffed Bell Peppers:

Ingredients:

Mini bell peppers

Cottage cheese or ricotta

Chopped herbs (parsley, basil)

Preparation: Stuff the mini bell peppers with cottage cheese or ricotta and sprinkle chopped herbs on top.

Fertility Benefits: Bell peppers are rich in antioxidants, and cottage cheese/ricotta provides protein and calcium.

RECIPE 12: Walnut Banana Bread:

Ingredients:

1 cup mashed bananas

1/4 cup honey

2 eggs

1 tsp vanilla extract

1 1/2 cups whole wheat flour

1/2 cup chopped walnuts

1 tsp baking powder

1/2 tsp baking soda

Pinch of salt

Preparation: Mix all the ingredients together and bake in a preheated oven at 350°F (175°C) for about 45 minutes.

Fertility Benefits: Walnuts are a great source of omega-3 fatty acids, and bananas offer vitamins and minerals important for fertility.

RECIPE 13: Carrot and Ginger Soup:

Ingredients:

4 large carrots, chopped

1-inch piece of fresh ginger, grated

1 onion, chopped

2 cups vegetable broth

1 cup coconut milk

Salt and pepper to taste

Preparation: In a pot, sauté onions and ginger. Add chopped carrots and vegetable broth. Cook until the carrots are tender. Blend the mixture with coconut milk, salt, and pepper.

Fertility Benefits: Carrots are rich in beta-carotene, while ginger has anti-inflammatory properties.

RECIPE 14: Fertility-Friendly Sushi Rolls:

Ingredients:

Sushi nori sheets

Cooked quinoa or brown rice

Avocado slices

Cooked shrimp or smoked salmon

Cucumber sticks

Pickled ginger and soy sauce (for dipping)

Preparation: Lay a nori sheet on a bamboo sushi mat. Spread a thin layer of quinoa or rice on the nori, leaving space at the edges. Add avocado, shrimp/salmon, and cucumber. Roll tightly using the bamboo mat. Slice and serve with pickled ginger and soy sauce.

Fertility Benefits: This sushi version is rich in nutrients like omega-3 fatty acids from seafood and healthy fats from avocado.

RECIPE 15: Blueberry Almond Bars:

Ingredients:

1 cup almonds

1 cup dried blueberries

1/4 cup honey

1/4 cup almond butter

1/2 tsp vanilla extract

Preparation: Blend almonds and dried blueberries in a food processor. Add honey, almond butter, and vanilla extract, then blend until combined. Press the mixture into a lined pan and refrigerate until firm. Cut into bars.

Fertility Benefits: Blueberries contain antioxidants, while almonds provide protein and healthy fats.

RECIPE 16: Sweet Potato Fries:

Ingredients:

Sweet potatoes, cut into fries

Olive oil

Paprika

Sea salt

Preparation: Toss sweet potato fries with olive oil, paprika, and sea salt. Bake in a preheated oven at 400°F (200°C) until crispy.

Fertility Benefits: Sweet potatoes are rich in beta-carotene, which converts to vitamin A, an essential nutrient for fertility.

RECIPE 17: Pomegranate Yogurt Parfait:

Ingredients:

Greek yogurt

Pomegranate seeds

Honey

Granola (optional)

Preparation: Layer Greek yogurt, pomegranate seeds, and drizzle honey. Add granola if desired.

Fertility Benefits: Pomegranate seeds are packed with antioxidants, which can support reproductive health.

RECIPE 18: Cocoa-Nut Energy Balls:

Ingredients:

1 cup dates (soaked)

1/2 cup shredded coconut

1/4 cup raw cacao powder

1/4 cup almonds

1 tbsp chia seeds

Preparation:

Blend all the ingredients in a food processor. Form the mixture into small balls.

Fertility Benefits: Cacao powder contains antioxidants, while dates and almonds provide essential nutrients.

RECIPE 19: Asparagus and Egg Salad:

Ingredients:

Steamed asparagus

Boiled eggs, sliced

Cherry tomatoes, halved

Balsamic vinaigrette dressing

Preparation:

Arrange steamed asparagus, sliced boiled eggs, and cherry tomatoes in a bowl. Drizzle with balsamic vinaigrette.

Fertility Benefits: Asparagus is a source of folate, while eggs offer essential proteins and nutrients.

RECIPE 20: Mixed Bean Salad:

Ingredients:

Mixed beans (black beans, chickpeas, kidney beans)

Red onion, finely chopped

Fresh cilantro, chopped

Lime juice

Olive oil

Salt and pepper to taste

Preparation:

Mix the beans, chopped onion, and cilantro. Dress with lime juice, olive oil, salt, and pepper.

Fertility Benefits: Beans are rich in fiber and protein, which can be beneficial for hormone balance and reproductive health.

CHAPTER 7:

Dessert Recipes

Boosting fertility and conception through diet can be influenced by various factors, including maintaining a healthy weight, getting proper nutrition, and ensuring a balanced diet rich in fertility-boosting nutrients. Here are dessert recipes with ingredients, preparation instructions, for women over 30:

RECIPE 1: Berry Yogurt Parfait
Ingredients:
Greek yogurt (full-fat): Provides calcium and probiotics that support reproductive health.
Mixed berries: Rich in antioxidants, vitamins, and fiber.

Honey: Contains natural sugars and can help regulate blood sugar levels.

Preparation:

Layer Greek yogurt and mixed berries in a glass. Drizzle honey on top.

RECIPE 2: Chia Seed Pudding

Ingredients:

Chia seeds: High in omega-3 fatty acids and fiber.

Almond milk: Contains Vitamin E and healthy fats.

Maple syrup: Adds natural sweetness and trace minerals.

Preparation:

Mix chia seeds and almond milk. Add maple syrup to sweeten. Refrigerate overnight until it thickens.

RECIPE 3: Dark Chocolate-Covered Strawberries

Ingredients:

Dark chocolate (70% cocoa or higher): Contains antioxidants and may boost blood flow.

Fresh strawberries: Rich in Vitamin C and folate.

Preparation:

Melt dark chocolate and dip strawberries in it. Let them cool on parchment paper.

RECIPE 4: Avocado Chocolate Mousse

Ingredients:

Avocado: High in healthy monounsaturated fats and Vitamin E.

Unsweetened cocoa powder: Rich in antioxidants.

Coconut milk: Provides healthy fats.

Preparation:

Blend avocado, cocoa powder, and coconut milk until smooth. Sweeten with honey if desired.

RECIPE 5: Banana Nut Muffins

Ingredients:

Ripe bananas: Contain Vitamin B6 and potassium.

Walnuts: Rich in omega-3 fatty acids and antioxidants.

Whole wheat flour: High in fiber and nutrients.

Preparation:

Combine mashed bananas, chopped walnuts, and whole wheat flour. Bake into muffins.

RECIPE 6: Pineapple Coconut Sorbet

Ingredients:

Fresh pineapple: Contains bromelain, an enzyme that may support implantation.

Coconut milk: Provides healthy fats.

Agave nectar: A natural sweetener.

Preparation:

Blend fresh pineapple and coconut milk. Sweeten with agave nectar. Freeze until firm.

RECIPE 7: Raspberry Almond Thumbprint Cookies

Ingredients:

Almond flour: High in Vitamin E and healthy fats.

Raspberries: Rich in antioxidants and Vitamin C.

Coconut oil: Contains healthy medium-chain triglycerides.

Preparation:

Mix almond flour and coconut oil. Form small balls, press a raspberry into each one, and bake.

RECIPE 8: Mango Lassi Popsicles

Ingredients:

Ripe mango: Rich in Vitamins A and C.

Greek yogurt (full-fat): Provides calcium and probiotics.

Preparation:

Blend mango and Greek yogurt until smooth. Pour into popsicle molds and freeze.

RECIPE 9: Cinnamon Baked Apples

Ingredients:

Apples: Contain Vitamin C and dietary fiber.

Cinnamon: May help regulate blood sugar levels.

Preparation:

Core apples and sprinkle with cinnamon. Bake until tender.

RECIPE 10: Pomegranate and Pistachio Dark Chocolate Bark

Ingredients:

Dark chocolate (70% cocoa or higher): Contains antioxidants and may boost blood flow.

Pomegranate seeds: Rich in antioxidants.

Pistachios: Provide healthy fats and protein.

Preparation:

Melt dark chocolate and spread it on parchment paper. Sprinkle pomegranate seeds and chopped pistachios on top. Let it cool and break into pieces.

RECIPE 11: Quinoa and Berry Parfait

Ingredients:

Cooked quinoa: High in protein and nutrients.

Mixed berries: Rich in antioxidants, vitamins, and fiber.

Greek yogurt (full-fat): Provides calcium and probiotics.

Preparation:

Layer cooked quinoa, mixed berries, and Greek yogurt in a glass.

RECIPE 12: Coconut Date Balls

Ingredients:

Dates: High in natural sugars and fiber.

Shredded coconut: Provides healthy fats.

Preparation:

Blend dates and shredded coconut until they form a sticky mixture. Roll into small balls.

RECIPE 13: Pumpkin Seed Brittle

Ingredients:

Pumpkin seeds: Rich in zinc and omega-3 fatty acids.

Honey: Contains natural sugars and can help regulate blood sugar levels.

Preparation:

Roast pumpkin seeds and drizzle with honey. Let them cool and harden.

RECIPE 14: Blueberry Oatmeal Bars

Ingredients:

Fresh blueberries: Rich in antioxidants and Vitamin C.

Rolled oats: High in fiber and nutrients.

Preparation:

Mix blueberries and rolled oats. Press into a baking dish and bake until set.

RECIPE 15: Orange Carrot Cake Bites

Ingredients:

Carrots: High in beta-carotene and fiber.

Almond flour: High in Vitamin E and healthy fats.

Oranges: Rich in Vitamin C.

Preparation:

Blend grated carrots, almond flour, and orange zest. Form into small balls.

RECIPE 16: Almond Butter Cups

Ingredients:

Almond butter: Provides healthy fats and protein.

Dark chocolate (70% cocoa or higher): Contains antioxidants and may boost blood flow.

Preparation:

Melt dark chocolate and fill the bottom of cupcake liners. Add a spoonful of almond butter and cover with more melted chocolate. Let them cool and set.

RECIPE 17: Spinach and Banana Smoothie

Ingredients:

Fresh spinach: Contains iron and folate.

Ripe bananas: Contain Vitamin B6 and potassium.

Greek yogurt (full-fat): Provides calcium and probiotics.

Preparation:

Blend spinach, bananas, and Greek yogurt until smooth.

RECIPE 18: Kiwi Lime Sorbet

Ingredients:

Kiwi: High in Vitamin C and antioxidants.

Lime juice: Contains Vitamin C.

Preparation:

Blend kiwi and lime juice. Freeze until firm.

RECIPE 19: Sesame Seed Energy Balls

Ingredients:

Sesame seeds: Rich in zinc and iron.

Dried apricots: Provide natural sweetness and fiber.

Preparation:

Blend sesame seeds and dried apricots until they form a sticky mixture. Roll into small balls.

RECIPE 20: Pear and Almond Crisp

Ingredients:

Pears: Contain Vitamin C and dietary fiber.
Almonds: High in Vitamin E and healthy fats.
Maple syrup: Adds natural sweetness and trace minerals.

Preparation:

Slice pears and place them in a baking dish. Sprinkle with chopped almonds and drizzle with maple syrup. Bake until tender.
These desserts are designed to include high fertility-boosting ingredients, they should still be consumed in moderation as part of a balanced diet.

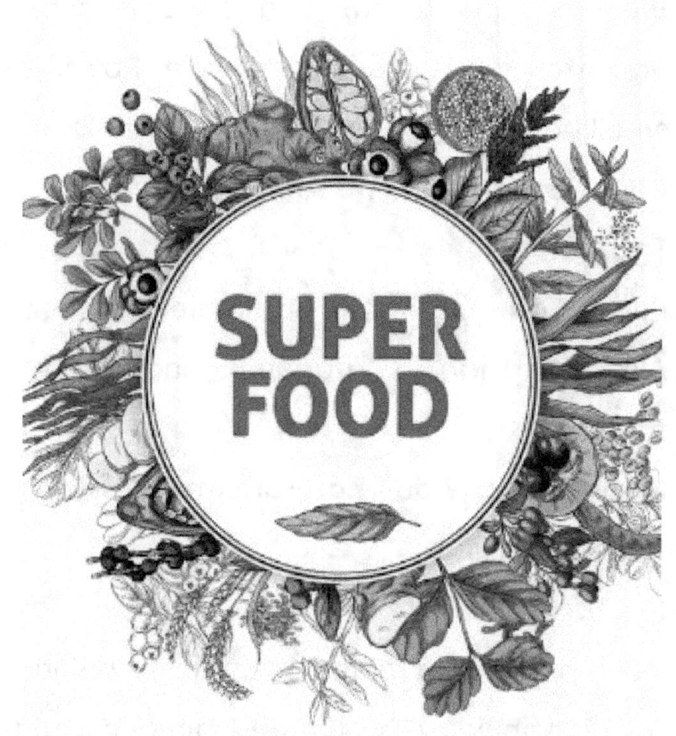

SUPER
FOOD

CHAPTER 8:

Special Drinks for Fertility

Fertility-Boosting Smoothie:

Fertility-boosting smoothies can be a delicious and nutritious way to support reproductive health. Below are smoothie recipes for women over 30, along with their ingredients, preparation, and fertility benefits:

RECIPE 1: Berry Blast

Ingredients:

1 cup mixed berries (blueberries, raspberries, strawberries)

1 banana

1 cup spinach

1 cup almond milk

Preparation: Blend all ingredients until smooth.

Fertility Benefits: Berries are rich in antioxidants and vitamin C, which may improve egg quality and overall fertility.

RECIPE 2: Green Goddess

Ingredients:

1 cup kale

1/2 cucumber

1/2 avocado

1/2 lemon (juiced)

1 cup coconut water

Preparation: Blend all ingredients until smooth.

Fertility Benefits: This green smoothie is loaded with vitamins, minerals, and healthy fats that support hormone balance and reproductive health.

RECIPE 3: Tropical Delight

Ingredients:

1 cup pineapple

1/2 mango

1 banana

1 cup coconut milk

Preparation: Blend all ingredients until smooth.

Fertility Benefits:

Pineapple contains bromelain, an enzyme that may aid implantation, while mango provides vitamin A, essential for reproductive function.

RECIPE 4: Golden Glow

Ingredients:

1 cup carrots (cooked and cooled)

1 orange (peeled)

1 inch fresh ginger (peeled)

1 cup water or orange juice

Preparation: Blend all ingredients until smooth.

Fertility Benefits:

Carrots are rich in beta-carotene, supporting healthy ovulation, while ginger has anti-inflammatory properties beneficial for fertility.

RECIPE 5: Almond Joy

Ingredients:

1 cup almond milk

2 tablespoons almond butter

1 tablespoon cacao powder

1 tablespoon honey

1/2 teaspoon vanilla extract

Preparation: Blend all ingredients until smooth.

Fertility Benefits: Almonds provide healthy fats and vitamin E, which may improve fertility and support reproductive tissues.

RECIPE 6: Chia-Cherry Bliss

Ingredients:

1 cup cherries (pitted)

1 tablespoon chia seeds

1 cup Greek yogurt

1 cup water or almond milk

Preparation: Blend all ingredients until smooth and let it sit for a few minutes to thicken.

Fertility Benefits: Chia seeds are rich in omega-3 fatty acids, supporting hormone production and reducing inflammation.

RECIPE 7: Spinach & Pineapple Paradise

Ingredients:

2 cups spinach

1 cup pineapple

1/2 banana

1 tablespoon flaxseed

1 cup coconut water or water

Preparation: Blend all ingredients until smooth.

Fertility Benefits:

Spinach offers iron and folic acid, essential nutrients for reproductive health, while flaxseed provides omega-3s and fiber.

RECIPE 8: Maca-Mango Magic

Ingredients:

1 cup mango

1 tablespoon maca powder

1 cup coconut milk

1 tablespoon honey (optional)

Preparation: Blend all ingredients until smooth.

Fertility Benefits: Maca is an adaptogenic herb that may help balance hormones and improve fertility in some women.

RECIPE 9: Raspberry Lemonade

Ingredients:

1 cup raspberries

1/2 lemon (peeled and seeded)

1 cup water or coconut water

1 tablespoon honey

Preparation: Blend all ingredients until smooth.

Fertility Benefits:

Raspberries contain antioxidants that support reproductive health, while lemon helps balance pH levels.

RECIPE 10: Pomegranate Power

Ingredients:

1 cup pomegranate seeds

1/2 cup Greek yogurt

1 banana

1 tablespoon honey

1 cup almond milk

Preparation: Blend all ingredients until smooth.

Fertility Benefits: Pomegranate seeds are rich in antioxidants and may improve blood flow to the uterus.

RECIPE 11: Apricot Sunrise

Ingredients:

1 cup apricots (pitted)

1/2 cup carrots (cooked and cooled)

1 tablespoon bee pollen (optional)

1 cup water or orange juice

Preparation: Blend all ingredients until smooth.

Fertility Benefits: Apricots provide vitamin A and iron, promoting fertility and healthy conception.

RECIPE 12: Kale & Kiwi Elixir

Ingredients:

1 cup kale

2 kiwis (peeled)

1 tablespoon hemp seeds

1 cup coconut water or water

Preparation: Blend all ingredients until smooth.

Fertility Benefits:

Kiwi is packed with vitamin C, which supports healthy ovulation, and kale offers essential vitamins and minerals.

RECIPE 13: Berry Avocado Boost

Ingredients:

1 cup mixed berries (strawberries, blueberries)

1/2 avocado

1 tablespoon flaxseed

1 cup almond milk

Preparation: Blend all ingredients until smooth.

Fertility Benefits: Avocado contributes healthy fats, while flaxseed provides omega-3s and fiber.

RECIPE 14: Turmeric Mango Magic

Ingredients:

1 cup mango

1/2 teaspoon turmeric

1/2 teaspoon cinnamon

1 cup coconut milk or water

Preparation: Blend all ingredients until smooth.

Fertility Benefits:

Turmeric has anti-inflammatory properties, and cinnamon may support healthy blood sugar levels.

RECIPE 15: Papaya Passion

Ingredients:

1 cup papaya

1 banana

1 cup coconut water or almond milk

1 tablespoon honey (optional)

Preparation: Blend all ingredients until smooth.

Fertility Benefits:

Papaya contains vitamins A and C, essential for reproductive health.

RECIPE 16: Blueberry Almond Dream

Ingredients:

1 cup blueberries

2 tablespoons almond butter

1 cup almond milk

1 tablespoon honey

Preparation: Blend all ingredients until smooth.

Fertility Benefits: Blueberries are rich in antioxidants and vitamins, supporting egg health and reproductive function.

RECIPE 17: Peachy Keen

Ingredients:

1 cup peaches (peeled and pitted)

1/2 cup Greek yogurt

1 tablespoon honey

1 cup water or almond milk

Preparation: Blend all ingredients until smooth.

Fertility Benefits: Peaches offer vitamin C and antioxidants, supporting reproductive health.

RECIPE 18: Beet Berry Blast

Ingredients:

1 cup beets (cooked and cooled)

1 cup mixed berries (raspberries, strawberries)

1 tablespoon honey

1 cup water or coconut water

Preparation: Blend all ingredients until smooth.

Fertility Benefits: Beets are rich in iron and nitrates, supporting blood flow and reproductive health.

RECIPE 19: Date & Walnut Wonder

Ingredients:

1 cup dates (pitted)

1/2 cup walnuts

1 cup almond milk

1/2 teaspoon vanilla extract

Preparation: Blend all ingredients until smooth.

Fertility Benefits: Dates and walnuts provide essential nutrients, including omega-3 fatty acids.

RECIPE 20: Mango-Coconut Bliss

Ingredients:

1 cup mango

1/2 cup shredded coconut

1 cup coconut milk

1 tablespoon honey

Preparation: Blend all ingredients until smooth.

Fertility Benefits: Mango and coconut offer essential vitamins and healthy fats for reproductive health.

Herbal Teas for Reproductive Health:

Herbal teas that are commonly believed to have potential benefits for women's fertility based on traditional knowledge.

RECIPE 1: Raspberry Leaf Tea:

Ingredients:

Dried raspberry leaves.

Preparation: Steep 1-2 teaspoons of dried raspberry leaves in hot water for 5-10 minutes.

Fertility Benefits: Raspberry leaf is believed to support uterine health and may help regulate menstrual cycles.

RECIPE 2: Nettle Tea:

Ingredients:

Dried nettle leaves.

Preparation: Steep 1-2 teaspoons of dried nettle leaves in hot water for 5-10 minutes.

Fertility Benefits: Nettle is rich in vitamins and minerals, which may support overall reproductive health.

RECIPE 3: Red Clover Tea:

Ingredients:

Dried red clover blossoms.

Preparation: Steep 1-2 teaspoons of dried red clover blossoms in hot water for 5-10 minutes.

Fertility Benefits: Red clover is thought to contain phytoestrogens, which might help balance hormone levels.

RECIPE 4: Dong Quai Tea:

Ingredients:

Dried dong quai root.

Preparation: Steep 1-2 teaspoons of dried dong quai root in hot water for 5-10 minutes.

Fertility Benefits: Dong quai is a traditional Chinese herb believed to support female reproductive health.

RECIPE 5: Chasteberry (Vitex) Tea:

Ingredients:

Dried chasteberry (Vitex) berries.

Preparation: Steep 1-2 teaspoons of dried chasteberry berries in hot water for 5-10 minutes.

Fertility Benefits: Chasteberry is believed to help regulate menstrual cycles and support hormonal balance.

RECIPE 6: Maca Root Tea:

Ingredients:

Maca root powder.

Preparation: Mix 1-2 teaspoons of maca root powder with hot water.

Fertility Benefits: Maca is thought to help balance hormones and support overall reproductive health.

RECIPE 7: Peony Tea:

Ingredients:

Dried peony root.

Preparation: Steep 1-2 teaspoons of dried peony root in hot water for 5-10 minutes.

Fertility Benefits: Peony is used in traditional Chinese medicine to support female fertility.

RECIPE 8: Dandelion Root Tea:

Ingredients:

Dried dandelion root.

Preparation: Steep 1-2 teaspoons of dried dandelion root in hot water for 5-10 minutes.

Fertility Benefits: Dandelion root is believed to support liver function and hormonal balance.

RECIPE 9: Cinnamon Tea:

Ingredients:

Cinnamon sticks or powder.

Preparation: Steep 1-2 cinnamon sticks or 1-2 teaspoons of cinnamon powder in hot water for 5-10 minutes.

Fertility Benefits: Cinnamon is believed to help regulate insulin levels, which may be beneficial for fertility.

RECIPE 10: Tribulus Terrestris Tea:

Ingredients:

Dried Tribulus Terrestris berries.

Preparation: Steep 1-2 teaspoons of dried Tribulus Terrestris berries in hot water for 5-10 minutes.

Fertility Benefits: Tribulus Terrestris is traditionally used to support female reproductive health.

RECIPE 11: False Unicorn Root Tea:

Ingredients:

Dried false unicorn root.

Preparation: Steep 1-2 teaspoons of dried false unicorn root in hot water for 5-10 minutes.

Fertility Benefits: False unicorn root is believed to support uterine health and hormonal balance.

RECIPE 12: Black Cohosh Tea:

Ingredients:

Dried black cohosh root.

Preparation: Steep 1-2 teaspoons of dried black cohosh root in hot water for 5-10 minutes.

Fertility Benefits: Black cohosh is believed to help regulate menstrual cycles and support reproductive health.

RECIPE 13: Ashwagandha Tea:

Ingredients:

Ashwagandha root powder.

Preparation: Mix 1-2 teaspoons of ashwagandha root powder with hot water.

Fertility Benefits: Ashwagandha is used in Ayurvedic medicine for its potential to support reproductive health.

RECIPE 14: Licorice Root Tea:

Ingredients:

Dried licorice root.

Preparation: Steep 1-2 teaspoons of dried licorice root in hot water for 5-10 minutes.

Fertility Benefits: Licorice root is thought to have anti-inflammatory properties that may support reproductive health.

RECIPE 15: Lemon Balm Tea:

Ingredients:

Fresh or dried lemon balm leaves.

Preparation: Steep 1-2 teaspoons of fresh or dried lemon balm leaves in hot water for 5-10 minutes.

Fertility Benefits: Lemon balm is believed to have calming properties that might be helpful during the fertility journey.

RECIPE 16: Passionflower Tea:

Ingredients:

Dried passion flower leaves.

Preparation: Steep 1-2 teaspoons of dried passion flower leaves in hot water for 5-10 minutes.

Fertility Benefits: Passionflower is thought to have relaxing properties that may support fertility health.

RECIPE 17: Oat Straw Tea:

Ingredients:

Dried oat straw.

Preparation: Steep 1-2 teaspoons of dried oat straw in hot water for 5-10 minutes.

Fertility Benefits: Oat straw is rich in nutrients that may be beneficial for reproductive health.

RECIPE 18: Lemon Verbena Tea:

Ingredients:

Fresh or dried lemon verbena leaves.

Preparation: Steep 1-2 teaspoons of fresh or dried lemon verbena leaves in hot water for 5-10 minutes.

Fertility Benefits: Lemon verbena is believed to have calming and soothing properties.

RECIPE 19: Ginseng Tea:

Ingredients:

Dried ginseng root.

Preparation: Steep 1-2 teaspoons of dried ginseng root in hot water for 5-10 minutes.

Fertility Benefits: Ginseng is thought to support reproductive health and boost energy levels.

RECIPE 20: Chamomile Tea:

Ingredients:

Fresh or dried chamomile flowers.

Preparation: Steep 1-2 teaspoons of fresh or dried chamomile flowers in hot water for 5-10 minutes.

Fertility Benefits: Chamomile is believed to have calming properties that might be beneficial for fertility.

Supplements and Superfoods :

Essential Vitamins and Minerals for Fertility:

Maintaining proper nutrition is essential for fertility in women over 30. Certain vitamins and minerals play a crucial role in supporting reproductive health. Here are some essential vitamins and minerals, their food sources, preparation tips, and their fertility benefits:

1). Folic Acid (Vitamin B9):

Food sources: Leafy greens (spinach, kale, collard greens), lentils, beans, fortified cereals, avocado.

Preparation: Consume these foods raw in salads or steamed for maximum nutrient retention.

Fertility benefits: Folic acid aids in the formation of the neural tube in the early stages of pregnancy, reducing the risk of neural tube defects in the baby. It also supports healthy ovulation and may improve egg quality.

2). Iron:

Food sources: Red meat, poultry, fish, lentils, spinach, tofu, fortified cereals.

Preparation: Cook meat and fish thoroughly. For vegetarian sources like lentils and spinach, cooking or steaming is recommended.

Fertility benefits: Iron helps maintain healthy blood hemoglobin levels, which are crucial for reproductive health. It enhances the chances of conceiving and reduces the risk of complications during pregnancy.

3). Vitamin D:

Food sources: Fatty fish (salmon, mackerel), fortified dairy products, egg yolks.

Preparation: Enjoy salmon and mackerel grilled or baked. For dairy products, consume them as they are or in smoothies.

Fertility benefits: Vitamin D is crucial for hormone regulation, including reproductive hormones. It may help improve fertility and support a healthy pregnancy.

4). Omega-3 Fatty Acids:

Food sources: Fatty fish (salmon, sardines, trout), chia seeds, flaxseeds, walnuts.

Preparation: Incorporate fish into your diet by baking, grilling, or poaching. Sprinkle chia seeds or ground flaxseeds on yogurt or salads.

Fertility benefits: Omega-3 fatty acids help regulate hormones and promote a healthy menstrual cycle. They also support a favorable uterine environment for conception and early pregnancy.

5). Zinc:

Food sources: Oysters, lean meats, beans, nuts, seeds, whole grains.

Preparation: Consume oysters and meats after proper cooking. For nuts and seeds, enjoy them as snacks or sprinkle on dishes.

Fertility benefits: Zinc is essential for proper cell division and DNA synthesis. It supports egg development and is vital for overall reproductive health.

6). Calcium:

Food sources: Dairy products (milk, yogurt, cheese), fortified plant-based milk, leafy greens.

Preparation: Consume dairy products or fortified plant-based milk as they are or use them in smoothies. Steam or sauté leafy greens.

Fertility benefits: Calcium is crucial for maintaining healthy uterine muscles and promoting proper embryo implantation.

Superfoods to Enhance Fertility:

Here's a list of superfoods, along with their ingredients, preparation, and fertility benefits:

1). Spinach:

Ingredients:

Fresh spinach leaves.

Preparation: Use raw in salads or lightly steam.

Fertility Benefits: Rich in iron and folate, which are essential for healthy ovulation and fetal development.

2). Avocado:

Ingredients:

Fresh avocado.

Preparation: Mash and spread on toast or use in salads.

Fertility Benefits: High in healthy fats, vitamin E, and potassium, which support hormonal balance and reproductive health.

3). Berries (Blueberries, Strawberries, Raspberries)

Ingredients:

Fresh or frozen berries

Preparation: Eat them as a snack or add to smoothies.

Fertility Benefits: Packed with antioxidants and vitamin C, which may improve egg quality.

4). Lentils:

Ingredients:

Dried lentils.

Preparation: Soak and cook according to instructions.

Fertility Benefits: A great source of plant-based protein and iron, promoting regular menstrual cycles.

5). Quinoa:

Ingredients:

Quinoa grains.

Preparation: Cook according to instructions.

Fertility Benefits: Contains essential amino acids, iron, and magnesium, which support reproductive health.

6). Walnuts:

Ingredients:

Raw walnuts.

Preparation: Eat them as a snack or add them to salads.

Fertility Benefits: Rich in omega-3 fatty acids, which may improve hormone production and reduce inflammation.

7). Sweet Potatoes:

Ingredients:

Fresh sweet potatoes.

Preparation: Roast or steam.

Fertility Benefits: High in vitamin A and antioxidants, supporting reproductive tissues and hormone balance.

8). Salmon:

Ingredients:

Fresh or wild-caught salmon.

Preparation: Grill or bake with light seasoning.

Fertility Benefits: A great source of omega-3 fatty acids and protein, which may enhance fertility.

9). Greek Yogurt:

Ingredients:

Plain Greek yogurt.

Preparation: Eat as is or add to smoothies.

Fertility Benefits: High in calcium and probiotics, promoting reproductive health and gut balance.

10). Chia Seeds:

Ingredients:

Chia seeds.

Preparation: Add to smoothies or soak in liquid to create chia pudding.

Fertility Benefits: Rich in omega-3 fatty acids and fiber, supporting hormonal function.

11). Broccoli:

Ingredients:

Fresh broccoli florets.

Preparation: Steam or roast lightly.

Fertility Benefits: Contains folate and vitamin C, supporting fertility and overall health.

12). Pumpkin Seeds:

Ingredients:

Raw pumpkin seeds.

Preparation: Eat as a snack or sprinkle on salads.

Fertility Benefits: Rich in zinc, which is crucial for reproductive hormone regulation.

13). Beans (Black Beans, Kidney Beans, Chickpeas):

Ingredients:

Canned or dried beans.

Preparation: Cook according to instructions or use canned varieties in recipes. Fertility Benefits: High in plant-based protein and fiber, supporting reproductive health.

14: Eggs:

Ingredients:

Organic, free-range eggs.

Preparation: Boil, poach, or scramble.

Fertility Benefits: A good source of high-quality protein and essential nutrients like choline, which may aid fertility.

15). Beets:

Ingredients:

Fresh beets.

Preparation: Roast, steam, or grate for salads.

Fertility Benefits: Rich in iron and nitrates, promoting blood flow and reproductive health.

16). Asparagus:

Ingredients:

Fresh asparagus spears.

Preparation: Roast, steam, or sauté lightly.

Fertility Benefits: Contains folate, vitamin C, and antioxidants, supporting fertility.

17). Brazil Nuts:

Ingredients:

Raw Brazil nuts.

Preparation: Eat as a snack.

Fertility Benefits: High in selenium, which may enhance fertility and thyroid function.

18). Oranges:

Ingredients:

Fresh oranges or freshly squeezed orange juice.

Preparation: Eat the fruit or drink the juice.

Fertility Benefits: Rich in vitamin C and antioxidants, promoting reproductive health.

19). Turmeric:

Ingredients: Turmeric powder or fresh turmeric root.

Preparation: Use in cooking or make golden milk with milk and honey.

Fertility Benefits: Contains curcumin, which may reduce inflammation and support fertility.

20). Dark Chocolate (70% cocoa or higher):

Ingredients:

Dark chocolate.

Preparation: Enjoy as a treat or use in recipes. Fertility Benefits: Contains antioxidants that may improve blood flow to the reproductive organs.

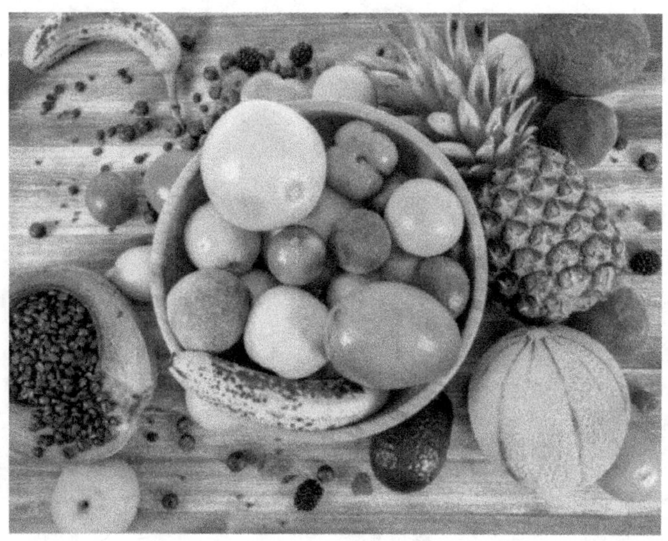

CHAPTER 9:

Lifestyle Tips for Boosting Fertility:

Boosting fertility in women over 30 can be influenced by various lifestyle factors. While age can affect fertility, there are steps women can take to optimize their chances of conceiving. Here are some lifestyle tips that may help:

Healthy Diet: Maintain a well-balanced diet rich in fruits, vegetables, whole grains, lean proteins, and healthy fats. Adequate intake of vitamins and minerals, such as folic acid, iron, and calcium, can support reproductive health.

Maintain a Healthy Weight: Being either underweight or overweight can affect fertility. Aim for a healthy weight range by engaging in regular physical activity and making appropriate dietary choices.

Quit Smoking: Smoking has a negative impact on fertility and can reduce the chances of conception. If you smoke, consider quitting to improve your reproductive health.

Limit Alcohol and Caffeine: Excessive alcohol and caffeine intake may interfere with conception. Consider reducing or eliminating these substances.

Stay Hydrated: Drink plenty of water to stay well-hydrated, as it can support overall health, including reproductive health.

Manage Stress: High levels of stress can affect hormones responsible for fertility. Practice stress-reduction techniques such as yoga, meditation, mindfulness, or engaging in hobbies you enjoy.

Exercise Regularly: Moderate and consistent exercise can help improve fertility and overall health. Avoid excessive and intense workouts, as they may have a negative impact on fertility.

Get Enough Sleep: Aim for 7-9 hours of quality sleep per night. Sufficient rest is crucial for hormone regulation and overall well-being.

Know Your Menstrual Cycle: Keep track of your menstrual cycle to identify the most fertile days for intercourse. There are various apps and tools available to help you track ovulation.

Preconception Checkup: Before trying to conceive, visit a healthcare provider for a preconception checkup. They can assess your overall health, provide valuable advice, and ensure any underlying health issues are addressed.

Avoid Exposure to Harmful Substances: Limit exposure to environmental toxins, hazardous chemicals, and certain medications that might interfere with fertility.

Consider Prenatal Vitamins: Taking prenatal vitamins with folic acid before conception can help reduce the risk of certain birth defects and support early fetal development.

Stay Informed: Stay informed about fertility and reproductive health. Knowledge empowers you to make informed decisions and seek professional help when necessary.

Exercise and Its Impact on Fertility:

Exercise can have both positive and negative impacts on fertility in women over 30. Let's explore these effects in more detail:

Positive Impact on Fertility:

Regular moderate exercise is generally beneficial for overall health, and it can positively affect fertility in some ways:

a. Hormonal Balance: Exercise can help regulate hormones such as insulin, cortisol, and thyroid hormones, which play a role in reproductive health.

b. Weight Management: Maintaining a healthy weight through exercise can be crucial for fertility. Obesity or being underweight can affect hormone production and ovulation.

c. Stress Reduction: Exercise is an excellent stress-reliever, and high levels of stress can interfere with reproductive hormones and ovulation.

d. Improved Circulation: Regular physical activity promotes better blood flow, which can be beneficial for reproductive organs.

e. Increased Endorphins: Exercise releases endorphins, which can positively influence mood and well-being, potentially benefiting fertility.

Negative Impact on Fertility: While moderate exercise is generally beneficial, excessive and intense exercise might have negative effects on fertility:

a. Irregular Menstrual Cycles: Intense exercise or excessive training can lead to irregular or absent menstrual cycles, known as hypothalamic amenorrhea. This hormonal imbalance can affect ovulation.

b. Overtraining and Stress: Too much exercise can cause physical stress on the body, leading to an increase in cortisol levels, which may disrupt reproductive hormones.

c. Low Body Fat: Intense exercise combined with inadequate calorie intake can lead to low body fat, which may negatively impact fertility by affecting hormone production.

d. Ovulatory Dysfunction: Some women may experience ovulatory dysfunction if they engage in excessive exercise, leading to difficulties in conceiving.

Individual Variations: It's important to note that the impact of exercise on fertility can vary significantly from one woman to another. While some women may experience improved fertility with moderate exercise, others may face challenges due to excessive exercise or other factors.

Exercise Routine For Fertility:

Here's a general exercise routine that can be beneficial for women over 30 who are trying to enhance their fertility:

Cardiovascular Exercise: Aim for at least 30 minutes of moderate-intensity cardio exercise most days of the week. This can include activities like brisk walking, jogging, swimming, or cycling. Cardiovascular exercise helps maintain a healthy weight and supports overall reproductive health.

Strength Training: Incorporate strength training exercises 2-3 times a week. Focus on compound movements that engage multiple muscle groups, such as squats, lunges, deadlifts, and push-ups. Strength training can help improve metabolism and hormone regulation.

Yoga and Stretching: Practice yoga or regular stretching exercises to improve flexibility, reduce stress, and promote relaxation. Stress can have a negative impact on fertility, so managing it through relaxation techniques is crucial.

Pelvic Floor Exercises: Strengthening the pelvic floor muscles can be beneficial for overall pelvic health. Kegel exercises can help improve pelvic tone and support reproductive organs.

Low-impact Exercises: Consider incorporating low-impact exercises like swimming or prenatal fitness classes.

These activities can be gentle on the body while still providing the benefits of exercise.

Mindfulness and Meditation: Engage in mindfulness practices and meditation to manage stress and support emotional well-being. High levels of stress can disrupt hormonal balance and potentially impact fertility.

Adequate Rest: Allow time for proper rest and recovery between exercise sessions. Quality sleep is essential for hormonal regulation and overall health.

Nutrition: Alongside exercise, maintain a balanced and nutritious diet. Ensure you're getting enough vitamins, minerals, and nutrients necessary for reproductive health, such as folate, iron, calcium, and omega-3 fatty acids.

Avoid Overtraining: Excessive exercise can potentially disrupt hormone levels. Strive for a moderate and balanced approach to your workout routine.

Stress Management Techniques:

Stress can have a significant impact on fertility, and women over 30 may experience increased stress due to various factors such as career demands, societal pressures, and concerns about fertility decline with age. Implementing stress management techniques can be beneficial for improving fertility in women over 30. Here are some strategies to consider:

Mindfulness and Meditation: Practicing mindfulness and meditation can help reduce stress and anxiety levels. Mindfulness involves being present in the moment and focusing on your thoughts and feelings without judgment. Regular meditation sessions can promote relaxation and a sense of calm.

Yoga: Yoga combines physical movement with breath control and meditation. It has been shown to reduce stress and improve overall well-being. Certain yoga poses can also target the reproductive system, potentially enhancing fertility.

Regular Exercise: Engaging in regular physical activity can help manage stress and improve overall health. Find an exercise routine that you enjoy, such as walking, jogging, swimming, or dancing, and aim for at least 30 minutes of moderate activity most days of the week.

Counseling or Therapy: Talking to a therapist or counselor can be helpful in addressing stress-related concerns and finding coping strategies specific to your situation.

Support Network: Build a support network of friends, family, or support groups with whom you can share your feelings and experiences. Sometimes, just talking to someone who understands can provide significant relief.

Time Management: Organize your daily activities and responsibilities to reduce feelings of being overwhelmed. Prioritize tasks and set realistic goals to manage your time effectively.

Relaxation Techniques: Incorporate relaxation techniques into your daily routine, such as deep breathing exercises, progressive muscle relaxation, or using calming essential oils.

Limit Information Overload: While it's essential to be informed about fertility, avoid overwhelming yourself with excessive information and stories from others. Set specific times to research and educate yourself about fertility, and then focus on other aspects of your life.

Limit Caffeine and Alcohol: Excessive caffeine and alcohol consumption can contribute to stress and affect fertility. Moderation is key.

Balanced Diet: A healthy, balanced diet can positively impact your overall well-being. Consider including fertility-friendly foods rich in antioxidants, vitamins, and minerals.

Prioritize Sleep: Ensure you get enough quality sleep each night as it plays a crucial role in managing stress and maintaining hormonal balance.

Creative Outlets: Engage in activities that allow you to express yourself creatively, such as painting, writing, or crafting.

Creative pursuits can serve as a form of therapy and relaxation.

The Importance of Sleep:

Sleep plays a crucial role in overall health and well-being, and its impact on fertility, especially in women over 30, cannot be overlooked. As women age, their fertility naturally starts to decline, and getting adequate sleep becomes even more important to support reproductive health. Here are some key reasons why sufficient sleep is essential for fertility in women over 30:

Hormone Regulation: Sleep is closely linked to hormonal regulation. Inadequate sleep can disrupt the delicate balance of hormones, including those involved in the menstrual cycle and ovulation, such as luteinizing hormone (LH) and follicle-stimulating hormone (FSH). Irregular or disrupted menstrual cycles can make it more challenging to predict the fertile window, which is crucial for conception.

Egg Quality: Quality eggs are essential for successful conception and a healthy pregnancy. Sleep deprivation and poor sleep quality can negatively impact egg quality. During sleep, the body goes through essential restorative processes, and this includes the repair and maintenance of cells, including eggs.

Stress Reduction: Chronic lack of sleep can increase stress levels, leading to the release of stress hormones like cortisol. Elevated cortisol levels can interfere with the production of reproductive hormones, potentially affecting ovulation and fertility.

Immune System Support: A well-functioning immune system is vital for maintaining a healthy reproductive system. Sleep helps strengthen the immune system, protecting against infections and inflammation that might affect fertility.

Weight Management: Adequate sleep is associated with better weight management. Sleep deprivation can disrupt hunger hormones like ghrelin and leptin, leading to increased appetite and potential weight gain. Being overweight or obese can negatively impact fertility in women.

Restoration and Recovery: Sleep provides the body with an opportunity to rest, recover, and repair. The reproductive system, like other bodily systems, requires sufficient rest to function optimally.

Regular Sleep Patterns: Establishing regular sleep patterns helps regulate the body's internal clock (circadian rhythm).

This consistency is essential for hormone balance and overall reproductive health.

Mental Health and Well-being: Sleep significantly influences mental health, and emotional well-being plays a crucial role in fertility. Chronic sleep deprivation can lead to mood disorders and increased stress levels, which may affect a woman's desire to conceive or her ability to cope with the challenges of trying to conceive.

Getting enough high-quality sleep is vital for fertility in women over 30. Aiming for 7-9 hours of sleep per night and practicing good sleep hygiene can contribute to improved hormonal balance, enhanced egg quality, reduced stress, and better overall reproductive health.

Fertility-Friendly Cooking Techniques

Fertility-friendly cooking techniques for women over 30 can help support reproductive health and optimize chances of conception.

Steaming: Steaming is a gentle cooking method that helps retain the nutrients in vegetables, such as folate and iron. Steam vegetables until they are just tender to preserve their fertility-boosting vitamins and minerals.

Sautéing: Use a small amount of healthy oil (like olive oil) to sauté vegetables and lean proteins. This method cooks food quickly, preserving nutrients, and adding healthy fats that are beneficial for hormone production.

Grilling: Grilling is a low-fat cooking technique that adds a delicious smoky flavor to food. Choose lean proteins like chicken, turkey, or fish and complement them with colorful vegetables for a nutrient-rich meal.

Baking: Baking is a great option for preparing fertility-friendly foods without excessive added fats. Try baking sweet potatoes, squash, or lean cuts of meat for a nutritious meal.

Poaching: Poaching eggs, chicken, or fish in water or broth can help retain their nutrients while avoiding added fats. This cooking method is gentle and keeps the food moist.

Stir-frying: Stir-frying quickly cooks vegetables and proteins, preserving their nutrients. Use minimal oil and add a variety of colorful vegetables for a nutrient-packed meal.

Raw and Fresh Foods: Include a variety of raw and fresh foods in your diet, such as salads with dark leafy greens, colorful vegetables, and fruits. These provide essential vitamins, minerals, and antioxidants.

Avoiding Overcooking: Overcooking foods can lead to nutrient loss. Try to cook foods until they are just tender to preserve their fertility-supporting properties.

Use Whole Foods: Opt for whole grains, such as brown rice and quinoa, which provide more nutrients and fiber compared to refined grains.

Hydration: Stay well-hydrated by drinking plenty of water throughout the day. Proper hydration is essential for overall health and may also support fertility.

Frequently Asked Questions

Can a gluten-free diet benefit fertility?

For people diagnosed with either gluten sensitivity or celiac disease. Incorporating a gluten-free diet into their lifestyle might prove beneficial for optimizing fertility outcomes. However, experts suggest that embracing this nutrition scheme isn't indispensable if you are free from these medical conditions and urge everyones' discretion in such matters.

Is it advisable to limit processed food consumption for fertility?

It is commonly suggested to restrict the consumption of processed foods for fertility as they usually contain harmful fats, sugars, and additives.

Does excessive sugar consumption impact fertility?

There is evidence indicating that a significant intake of refined sugars and sugary beverages may harm a person's fertility. It is suggested that limiting consumption of such products be considered to promote healthy reproductive function.

Can a Mediterranean diet support fertility?

Studies have shown that people who follow a Mediterranean-style diet consisting of fruits, vegetables, whole grains and good fats like fish can potentially experience enhanced fertility outcomes.

Does weight affect fertility?

When it comes to fertility one should keep in mind that both being underweight or overweight could potentially pose problems. Thus ensuring a healthy weight is critical to maintaining optimal reproductive health.

Is it beneficial to consume seafood for fertility?

Seafood - particularly high-fat fish like salmon and sardines - is an ideal dietary cornerstone for those seeking to enhance their reproductive health.

Is banana good for conceiving?

Rich sources of potassium and vitamin B6 in bananas help to improve sperm and egg quality thereby increasing fertility.

Fertility Weekly Meal Plan

	Breakfast	Lunch	Snacks	Dinner
Monday	Yogurt, granola, fresh berries	Fish tacos with spicy grilled veg salsa	Pomegranate juice, oatmeal cookies	Sardines and sauteed spinach with garlic
Tuesday	Steel cut oatmeal, walnuts, shaved coconut	Oysters, potatoes with mature cheese	Dry fruit ice cream with cinnamon dust	Raw oysters with 2-3 drops of lemon
Wednesday	Pancakes with shaved coconut, almond	Half cup cottage cheese, pumpkin seeds smoothie	Baked yams and cheese	Quinoa with leafy greens and tomatoes
Thursday	Scrambled egg bake, banana smoothie	Brown rice with chicken and yogurt raita	Citrus ice cream with figs and nuts	Beans and lentils curry with roti
Friday	Special salad with fruits and nuts	Garlic rice, roasted asparagus, and	Seaweed pasta with sesame seeds	Pancakes with honey and berries
Saturday	Egg toast, avocadoes, and sweet potatoes	Roasted red pepper, spinach puree	Roasted Meat with feta cheese and leafy greens	Walnuts and sunflower snacks with mature cheese
Sunday	Tomato soup, salmon fry	Mixed fruit smoothie, banana pancakes	Maca root with extra virgin olive oil dressing	Roasted sardines, yam with tomato sauce

Maintain a healthy weight and exercise regularly

DO'S	DON'TS
Increase intake of fruits and vegetables rich in vitamin C, fiber, folic acid, antioxidants, and nutrients	Avoid soy and soy products like soymilk, tofu
Taking multivitamins	More coffee consumption
Prefer organic dairy, fruits, and vegetables	Never consider genetically modified foods like GM corn and soy
Take required amounts of fat to improve hormone balance	Avoid refined and processed foods as they lead to hormone imbalance
Take a good amount of fiber to remove excess fat and hormones	Stop using plastic material items like bottles
Include essential proteins through lean proteins like chicken	Avoid eating red meat like tuna steak, and shark
Quit smoking, drugs, and alcohol consumption	Maintain a healthy weight and exercise regularly

CHAPTER 10:

The Connection Between Spirituality And Pregnancy

Spirituality and pregnancy are interconnected in various ways for many individuals. Pregnancy can be a transformative and profound experience, leading some people to explore their spiritual beliefs and practices more deeply. For some, the process of creating and nurturing new life can evoke feelings of awe, wonder, and connection to a higher power or universal energy. Spirituality during pregnancy may involve seeking guidance, finding comfort, or seeking a sense of purpose and meaning.

Many cultures have spiritual rituals and traditions surrounding pregnancy, childbirth, and motherhood, which can play a significant role in providing support and a sense of community during this transformative time. Some expectant parents may turn to prayer, meditation, or mindfulness practices to cope with the physical and emotional changes that come with pregnancy.

Some spiritual beliefs and practices focus on the idea of the soul or spirit entering the developing fetus, adding another layer of significance to the journey of pregnancy.

Spirituality during pregnancy can vary greatly from person to person, and not everyone may experience or embrace it in the same way. Although each individual's beliefs and experiences are unique and personal.

Spiritual Meditations And Prayers For Promoting Pregnancy.

Meditation and prayers may be helpful for some individuals during pregnancy, here are some spiritual meditations and prayers that some people find comforting:

Meditation for Peace and Relaxation: Sit in a comfortable position, close your eyes, and take deep breaths. Visualize a warm, comforting light surrounding you and your partner, fostering a sense of peace and relaxation. Focus on letting go of any stress or anxiety related to pregnancy.

Prayer for Fertility: Offer a prayer to your chosen higher power, seeking guidance and blessings for fertility and conception. Express your hopes and desires with sincerity and humility.

This involves entirely on what you believe in or your cultural practices.

Whether you are a Christian, Muslim, or whatever deity you believe in.

Gratitude Meditation: Practice a meditation of gratitude, where you express thanks for the blessings in your life, including the opportunity to create a family.

Visualization for Conception: Visualize a healthy and happy pregnancy, imagining yourself and your partner lovingly nurturing a baby in your arms. This is one principle that has worked for many who desire to conceive. Your mind pulls to you whatever you imagine or visualize, so you could put this to work by always visualizing yourself being pregnant, you stand in front of a mirror and visualize yourself while speaking to yourself saying something like *"I am pregnant"!*.

Prayer for Strength: Pray for the strength to navigate any challenges or difficulties you may encounter on your journey to parenthood.

Connection with Nature: Spend time in nature, whether it's in a garden or a peaceful outdoor setting. Allow the natural world to bring you a sense of renewal and connection.

__Thanks For Reading Every Piece!!!!__